GW00458143

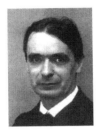

RUDOLF STEINER (1861–1925) called his spiritual philosophy 'anthroposophy', meaning 'wisdom of the human being'. As a highly developed seer, he based his work on direct knowledge and perception of spiritual dimensions. He initiated a modern and universal 'science of spirit', accessible to anyone willing to exercise clear and unprejudiced thinking.

From his spiritual investigations Steiner provided suggestions for the renewal of many activities, including education (both general and special), agriculture, medicine, economics, architecture, science, philosophy, religion and the arts. Today there are thousands of schools, clinics, farms and other organizations involved in practical work based on his principles. His many published works feature his research into the spiritual nature of the human being, the evolution of the world and humanity, and methods of personal development. Steiner wrote some 30 books and delivered over 6000 lectures across Europe. In 1924 he founded the General Anthroposophical Society, which today has branches throughout the world.

GOOD HEALTH

SELF-EDUCATION AND
THE SECRET OF WELL-BEING

RUDOLF STEINER

Compiled and introduced by Harald Haas

Translated by Matthew Barton

RUDOLF STEINER PRESS

Rudolf Steiner Press,
Hillside House, The Square
Forest Row, RH18 5ES

www.rudolfsteinerpress.com

Published by Rudolf Steiner Press 2017

Originally published in German under the title *Sich selbst erziehen* by
Rudolf Steiner Verlag, Basel, in 2014

A catalogue record for this book is available from the British Library

Print book ISBN: 978 1 85584 533 6
Ebook ISBN: 978 1 85584 492 6

Cover by Morgan Creative featuring image © eplisterra
Typeset by DP Photosetting, Neath, West Glamorgan
Printed and bound by 4Edge Ltd., Essex

Contents

Introduction:
The Basic Ideas Behind Salutogenesis   1
by Harald Haas

Forgetting   11
Berlin, 2 November 1908

Seminar Discussions on the Temperaments   27
Stuttgart, August 1919

Self-education   30
Berlin, 14 March 1912

For the Days of the Week   58

Notes   63

Sources   65

Introduction

THE BASIC IDEAS BEHIND SALUTOGENESIS

In Rudolf Steiner's pedagogical lectures he tells us repeatedly that education and health have been seen as connected from time immemorial:

> The idea was that when a person is born into earthly existence, he is really one level lower than truly human, and that he must first be drawn up, educated up, healed up to the human level. Education was seen as healing, was intrinsically part of medicine and healthcare.[1]

One of the primary endeavours of Rudolf Steiner's pedagogy was to reconnect these two fields, in practical terms through the collaboration of teachers with the school doctor. It was important to him that:

> ...education can only be rightly practised if it is regarded as curative, if the teacher is aware that he must be a healer.[2]

In ancient times, self-education was also called 'self-cultivation',[3] and seen as something vital to health in adult life. In his book 'Salutogenesis—Towards Health'[4] (in the chapter entitled 'Self-Education and the Cultivation of Health') Marco Bischof gives a survey of this ancient outlook. He also traces how the same theme, originating in ancient and eastern wisdom, was taken up again by modern philosophers such as Michel Foucault, Gernot Böhme and Peter Sloterdijk.

In the works of Rudolf Steiner, too, we find countless comments about 'self-development', not only as it relates to acquiring faculties of supersensible cognition but also as a way of improving health and coping better with ordinary life.

The texts compiled in this volume aim to present some basic ideas on education and self-education in connection with health and illness, (salutogenesis or hygiogenesis, as it is now called, and pathogenesis). It is astonishing that the concept of salutogenesis, first formulated in the 70s of the last century by the American-Israeli medical sociologist Aaron Antonovsky, has so quickly become current in a range of medical fields. While it seems a new paradigm, closer scrutiny actually shows it to have many, much older antecedents.

Rudolf Steiner's account of the whole context of human health and illness still goes far beyond ordinary scientific views, since alongside physical aspects he also includes soul-spiritual ones that come to expression in questions of destiny and repeated lives on earth. Two lectures from 1908 and 1912 were chosen as fundamental statements on these themes, extended and enlarged by extracts from other works by Steiner.

The first lecture, 'Forgetting' (in GA 107), was given to members of the Berlin branch of the Theosophical Society on 2 November 1908, and focuses primarily on memory as the basis of education and cultural development as well as its significance for health and illness. It also picks up on aspects of after-death existence and, at the end, characterizes the temperaments and their importance for health.

In the public lecture Steiner gave on 14 March 1912, 'Human Self-education in the Light of Spiritual Science' (in GA 61), Steiner presents self-education as a schooling of the will, and distinguishes it from the training of thought life. Elements that surface here are free play and gymnastics as well as empathy, conscience, and the cultivation of certain fundamental ideas through to the acceptance of destiny.

Below, by way of introduction, I will briefly outline and discuss the basic ideas contained in these lectures.

The lecture on 'Forgetting', which self-evidently considers both memory and the process of remembering, starts with our ordinary daily experiences of these. Memory is here shown to be located in the etheric body, while the astral body is seen as responsible for providing impressions and stimulus. Unlike the plant, part of the human being's etheric body is free, and it is here that education can exert an informing influence by developing soul-spiritual qualities. By contrast, what we bring with us as inherited characteristics is incorporated into our physical, etheric and soul corporeality as habits, passions and instincts. In other words, aspects of heredity and education interpenetrate in the various levels or 'bodies' of our human nature. Only in the free part of the etheric body can new ideas enter us through education and contribute to our cultural development.

People certainly vary a great deal in their capacity to absorb and assimilate new ideas. Rudolf Steiner assumes that someone who is more flexible in this regard will find it easier to engage in processes of healing or, in modern terminology, will have better capacities of salutogenesis.

Steiner goes on to show that in our conscious life of

thought, forgetting is a wholesome ability since, for example, being unable to forget anxieties and hurts or slights will in turn damage health. But in a more far-reaching stratum of the memory, all memories are retained. After death they are experienced as a memory tableau lasting several days, as is well known from accounts of near-death experiences. In the after-death period of kamaloka (Sanskrit = place of desires; or purgatory in Christian terminology) negative memories are distinguished from positive ones, and the latter, as the achievements and fruits of the life that is past, become the 'shapers and crafters' (Rudolf Steiner) of our next life. Here our memories are no longer dependent on an individual etheric body, which has by now largely dissolved into the universal ether, but are instead available to our soul and spirit through all that is inscribed in the Akashic Records, as they are known, in which memory is retained of everything that happens in the world.

A brief account of the temperaments as enduring characteristics rooted in the etheric body shows how people of different temperaments relate very differently to thoughts. In the sanguine and phlegmatic, they 'evaporate swiftly' (Steiner) and thus sustain health, whereas the melancholic 'simply cannot get beyond certain thoughts' (Steiner) and thereby greatly burdens his health. On the basis of this outlook we can form moral ideas, emancipated from egoism, founded solely on ideas of the human soul and spirit. The qualitative differentiation of temperaments in this lecture lays the ground for all of Rudolf Steiner's later ideas about education.

Two short sections from the 'seminar discussions' of August 1919 (in GA 295) develop these ideas about the temperaments, showing that they work right into a child's bodily form. Like the other three, the choleric temperament should be seen as a positive capacity. The temperaments can however assume extreme forms that come close to mental illness. Here Steiner employs Aristotelian concepts of madness, idiocy, imbecility and mania which are no longer current in our categories of illness.[5]

In the lecture 'Human Self-education in the Light of Spiritual Science', Steiner first distinguishes between the development of supersensible capacities of perception—which are not the concern here—and self-education for ordinary life. Appended here is a reference to *The Education of the Child in the Light of Spiritual Science* (in GA 34), in which, in 1907, Steiner had previously outlined his pedagogical principles. As opposed to education in childhood, as adults we become our own educators.

Careful study of the structure of the following lecture shows it to be arranged according to the principles of the path of mindfulness, as Gautama Buddha originally established it. Because of its eight stages or levels, it is called the 'eightfold path' or also the 'path of compassion'. Various accounts by Steiner engage with and renew this Buddhist path. It appears as the 'path of knowledge' in *Theosophy* (GA 9) and as 'development of the throat chakra' in *Knowledge of the Higher Worlds* (GA 10) as well as in exercises for each day of the week in *Soul Exercises* (GA 267, SteinerBooks 2015). To offer orientation about the contents of this path of practice, the exercises 'For the Days of the Week' are appended here as a final text .

For a clearer overview, marginal notes referring to each

step on the eightfold path can be found in the text on 'Self-education': our stance towards other people and the world (p. 33) as *right opinion*; an open mind as *right judgement* (p. 34); personal sympathy (p. 35) as *false judgement*; sympathy compassion, encompassing love (p. 36) and impulses of conscience (p. 37) as *right action*; gymnastic games (p. 41) as *right standpoint*; the education of the will in and through life (p. 42) as *human striving*; concentration and the assimilation of thoughts into a few fundamental ideas (p. 49) and learning to forget (p. 52) in order to improve mindfulness and imagination as *right memory*; and, finally, acceptance of our destiny (p. 54) as *right contemplation*.

From this list it becomes apparent that all aspects of the exercises 'For the Days of the Week' are contained in this lecture, in the proper sequence. We can therefore assume that Rudolf Steiner's method of self-education corresponds to that of the eightfold path.

In his account of aspects of self-education, great value is also placed on free play as right deed, as well as on gymnastic play as a form of self-education. This may remind us of Friedrich Schiller who, in his *Letters on the Aesthetic Education of Man*, accentuated the importance of play. In Letter 15 he writes:

> And so, to express it in full clarity for once, we can say that the human being plays only when he is human in the full sense of the word, and is only fully human when he plays.

In a later era—in the book *One-Dimensional Man* (1967)— Herbert Marcuse, among others, took up the idea of *Homo ludens* (a term coined by Johan Huizinga in his book of that name published in 1938/39).

What Steiner calls gymnastic play in this lecture eventually came to expression in the art of eurythmy from 1912 onwards. In subsequent years Steiner developed it further in artistic, educational and therapeutic directions.

On page 52 of the lecture on self-education, the theme of forgetting which figured in the first lecture is taken up again. Here too Steiner elaborates on the beneficial effect on our soul life of forgetting inessential thoughts, feelings, pain and suffering. This capacity to forget, above all, sustains mindfulness, attentiveness and imagination as a 'fertilizing, enlivening and life-enhancing element'. These two accounts of the health-giving benefits of a capacity for forgetting play into each other very harmoniously.

Towards the end of the lecture on self-education, Steiner mentions the phenomenon of nervousness and describes it as a miseducation of the will. He emphasizes that the will can only be educated through engagement with life and not by intellectual methods that act only on the life of thinking. At the beginning of 1912, on 11 January in Berlin, Steiner had already given exercises for overcoming nervousness, in a lecture to members entitled 'Nervousness and I-hood' (published in English as *How to Cure Nervousness*, Rudolf Steiner Press).

If we compare the exercises given there with the elements of the eightfold path and the exercises for the days of the week, we find a great affinity between them, but presented in the reverse sequence. In *How to Cure Nervousness* Steiner begins with an exercise to remedy forgetfulness ('right memory') followed by others against fidgetiness ('human striving'), inattentiveness ('right standpoint'), lack of form ('right deed'), weakness of will ('right speech'), indecisiveness ('right judgement') and finally presumptuousness ('right opinion'). Right contemplation can be found in the 'reality of spiritual-scientific understanding'.[6]

Rudolf Steiner's thoughts on reincarnation and karma are also relevant to the theme of nervousness. Another volume in this series on that subject[7] contains an article which Steiner published in 1906, entitled 'How health and illness relate to the law of karma'. There alongside the four temperaments he mentions a fifth that leads to nervousness:

> A life led thoughtlessly leads in a subsequent life to a shallow or happy-go-lucky predisposition which manifests particularly in forgetfulness and poor memory; and in a further life this forgetfulness appears as a potentially pathological condition which today is commonly called 'nervousness'.

My own clinical experience has taught me that nervousness does indeed appear as a fifth quality alongside other temperaments, and in a sense independently of them. The thought-devoid life of modern times, which leads to an increasing incidence of nervous conditions, can be seen as the outcome of dominant intellectual and materialistic outlooks. In other words, it is our modern destiny. This does not mean, however, that nothing should be done about it. As cited above, in various texts Steiner recommended the exercises of the eightfold path to overcome the modern disease of nervousness. Today, in fact, forms of treatment based on mindfulness, drawing on Buddhist teachings, are increasingly used in psychotherapy and even, recently, in schools.

To conclude I would like to highlight three key qualities from the lecture 'Self-education', upon which is based the 'whole spiritual-scientific outlook ... that we can to some degree get beyond ourselves, beyond what is enclosed within the confines of our personality, but without losing ourselves in the process'. Two elements are first mentioned here: sympathy and conscience. But then, at the end of the lecture, Steiner speaks of the possibility of 'repeatedly leading the sum of thoughts, emotions and perceptions back to a few basic ideas'. This can also be described as a mood of reverence or wonder. Steiner continually referred to these three capacities, of wonder, sympathy and conscience, in lectures he gave in various places at the end of 1911 and in the first half of 1912. He saw them as essential elements through which we can connect with the world of spirit and especially with the workings of Christ.[8]

Besides their spiritual effect, these three qualities are also very useful in the therapeutic and especially the psychotherapeutic domain. It would be reasonable to claim that a healthy, salutogenetic psychotherapy would work primarily with these elements: wonder, leading to real understanding of another's life situation, sympathy and empathy, and lastly conscience, in terms of the therapist's own 'authenticity' and integrity. The self-education of those seeking help and healing should involve their developing ability to gain understanding of their situation and relate to it reverently; to meet their fellow human beings with sympathy; and to find meaning and purpose in life through reconciliation with their destiny. This lecture on self-education is a stimulus for such work, a prerequisite for an anthroposophically oriented psychotherapy which seeks to help patients engage and connect with their earthly aims.

As Steiner himself predicted in his concluding remarks in the lecture, in relation to comments by Arthur Schopenhauer and Lessing, we are still only beginning to take up his suggestions and realize them in the modern world. Today, a century after this lecture was given, we can endeavour to develop things in this direction. It is clear from books on philosophical questions of self-development that I referred to earlier, that there is keen interest in such an undertaking.

Harald Haas
Bern, March 2012

Forgetting

BERLIN, 2 NOVEMBER 1908

Today we will embark on one of those spiritual-scientific trains of enquiry that show us how knowledge we can acquire through the anthroposophic world-view can illumine life in the broadest sense. Nor is it only ordinary, everyday life that becomes more comprehensible through such knowledge, for it also gives us insights of far-reaching scope as we seek to look beyond this life and penetrate what happens in the periods of our existence between death and a new birth. But spiritual science is assuredly also of great benefit for our daily life: it can solve certain enigmas and show us how we can cope better with our lives. You see, someone who is unable to fathom the depths of existence fails to understand things that happen to him every day, indeed, every hour. Many questions rise up in him which sense perception cannot answer and which, if they remain unanswered, become a hindrance in life, a cause of dissatisfaction. Dissatisfaction can never serve a person's development nor have a salutary effect on humanity. There are hundreds of such enigmas, and solving them can shed a much more profound light on life than we commonly imagine.

The word 'forgetting' conceals many such enigmas. You all know it as the word which indicates the opposite of retention of a certain thought or impression. No doubt all of you have been troubled to experience what this word means.

You will all have been disconcerted to discover that a certain idea, a certain impression has 'vanished' from your mind. And then you may have wondered why forgetting seems to be intrinsic to our experience of life.

In fact we can only gain useful insight into this question by drawing on occult realities. As you know, the mind, the memory, is connected with what we call the human etheric body. And so we can assume that the opposite of memory, forgetting, will also have something to do with the etheric body. We have to ask this: Is there some reason why we are able to forget things we once knew? Or should we make do with the common negative assumption that this failure to retain everything at every moment is a kind of deficiency of the soul? We will only gain insight into forgetting when we consider the importance of its opposite, the significance and nature of memory.

If we say that our memory has something to do with the human etheric body, we also have to ask why it falls to the etheric body to retain impressions and ideas. After all, the plant also has an etheric body, and there it has a substantially different task. We have often discussed the fact that the substance of a plant before us, compared to an inert stone, is permeated entirely by its etheric body. In the plant, the etheric body is the life principle in the narrower sense, and then also the principle of repetition. If the plant were subject only to the activity of the etheric body, it would put forth only leaf after leaf from the root upwards. It is due to the etheric body that parts and limbs continually recur, since it always seeks to produce the same thing again and again. Reproduction is also due to this—the reproducing of one's own kind. That too is based on an activity of the etheric body. Everything in us and in animals that depends on recurrence can be traced back to the etheric principle. The fact that vertebra after vertebra is repeated in the spine depends on this activity of the etheric body. But the fact that a plant's growth ends above in the flower, as a culmination of its vegetative existence, is due to another principle: to the earth's astrality entering the plant from without. Likewise, the fact that our vertebrae expand above to form hollow structures and the skull is due to the activity of the human being's astral body. Everything that creates conclusions, an end to growth, is subject to the astral, while all repetition originates in the etheric principle. The plant has this etheric body, and we human beings do too. Naturally the plant has no memory. It would be far-fetched to say—although modern science tends in that direction—that a plant possesses a kind of unconscious memory,[9] and notices what the leaf was like that it just put forth, then creates another such according to the same model. People even say that heredity can be attributed to a kind of unconscious memory. This is actually causing some mischief in scientific literature, for to speak of memory in the case of the plant is really shallow and inept.

The etheric body embodies the principle of repetition. But now, to grasp the difference between the etheric body in the plant and in the human being, in the latter case its capacity, alongside characteristics typical of the plant, to develop the memory also, we have to understand how plant and human being are distinct from each other in general. If you plant a seed in the ground, a quite specific plant grows from it. A wheat seed grows into a wheat stalk and ears of wheat while a bean produces a bean plant. And you will be compelled to say that the way in which each plant develops is unalterably determined by the nature of its seed. It is true that a gardener may come and transform or refine the plant through grafting perhaps or various other horticultural arts. But basically that is an exceptional situation and anyway of small scope compared with the inherent tendency of a plant to grow in a certain way and assume a particular form. Is this also true of us? Yes, to a certain degree—but no further than that. When a human being develops from the embryo we see that he too meets certain limits and constraints in his development. Black parents will have a black child, white parents a white one, and a whole range of other characteristics could be cited to show that human development, like that of the plant, is confined within certain parameters. But this is true only up to a certain point—it affects our physical, etheric and also astral nature. In the habits and impulses of the child we will be able to discern things similar to those of his ancestors, and these qualities will remain in him throughout life. But if we were as constrained by the limits of a certain type of growth as the plant is, there would be no such thing as education, the development of qualities of sensibility and mind. If you imagine two children of different parents, whose potential and outward characteristics are very similar, and then picture one of them being sorely neglected, given little education, while the other is carefully raised, sent to a good school and helped to develop all kinds of abilities, it is impossible to say that this development was already contained and fore-shadowed in the child's embryo in the same way that the bean plant is prefigured in the bean. The bean will grow whatever happens and does not need to be educated. That's its nature. We can't educate plants but we can educate human beings. We can pass knowledge on, or down, to people, introduce something into them which we cannot do in the same way in the case of the plant. Why is this? It is because the plant's etheric body always has a certain intact inner pattern which develops from one seed to the next within confines that cannot be exceeded. The human etheric body is different. Here, besides the part of the etheric body used for growth, for the kind of development which we have in common with the plant and within which we are similarly confined, there is another freely manifesting part that has no predetermined use if, through education, we do not teach a person— incorporate into his soul—all kinds of things that this free part of the etheric body subsequently assimilates. There really is in us, therefore, a part of the etheric body that nature does not employ. We do not use it for growth, for our natural organic development, but we retain is as a free element within us through which we can take up and absorb the ideas that enter us through education.

But now this absorption of ideas occurs initially through the impressions we receive. We always have to receive impressions, and all education depends on impressions and on the interplay between the etheric and astral body. To receive impressions we need the astral body. But to retain the impression so that it does not simply vanish again the etheric body is needed. For the slightest, seemingly insignificant memory the activity of the etheric body is required. For instance, if you look at an object the astral body is necessary for this. But to retain an image of it when you turn your head away the etheric body is needed. The astral body is involved in looking at something while the picture or idea of it requires the etheric body. Even though the degree of activity of the etheric body is very limited here, and though it really only comes fully into play where enduring habits, enduring inclinations, changes of temperament and so forth arise, nevertheless the etheric body is needed here already. It has to be there even if only to retain a simple idea in the mind, for all retention of ideas depends to some degree on memory.

Having incorporated all kinds of things into the free part of a person's etheric body through 'educational impressions', through development of his faculties, we can now ask this: does this free etheric element have no significance at all for the person's growth and physical development? No, that is not the case. Gradually as we grow older—not so much in our youth—what was incorporated into our etheric body through the impressions we received in our education starts to participate in the whole life of the human body, also inwardly. You can best comprehend this participation if I tell you something that people usually do not consider in ordinary life. They tend to think that our inner sensibility is not generally all that important in life. And yet the following can happen. Imagine that someone falls ill simply because he was exposed to unfavourable climatic conditions. We have to hypothesize that his illness can be affected by two possible conditions: firstly by the fact that he does not have much to assimilate in the free part of his etheric body. Let's assume he's a lethargic fellow upon whom the outer world makes little impression, who posed a considerable obstacle for educational efforts, someone for whom things go in one ear and out the other. Such a person will not have the same means of regaining his health as another who has a lively, vivid sensibility, who absorbed many things in his youth, assimilated many things, and therefore took very good care of the free part of his etheric body. The external focus of mainstream medicine has so far prevented it from discovering why one person heals more easily than another. This free element in the etheric body, energized through its manifold impressions, here comes into play and participates in the healing process by virtue of its inner mobility. In numerous instances people owe their quick or painless recovery to the fact that in their youth they industriously absorbed the impressions presented to them with lively mental and spiritual involvement. Here you see the influence of the mind or spirit on the body. Recovery is a quite different matter in someone who passes dully through life as compared to someone whose free etheric body does not stay ponderous and lethargic but vital and responsive. You just have to observe things with an open mind and then you will see how illnesses affect people differently, depending on whether they are mentally lethargic or lively and responsive.

And so you can see that the human etheric body is very different from that of the simple plant. The plant lacks this free part of the etheric body which we humans can develop. In fact our whole human evolution depends really on the fact that we possess this free etheric component. If you compare beans of a millennium ago with modern beans, you will discern a certain difference but really a very small one. The beans have broadly retained their form. But if you compare Europeans at the time of Charlemagne with modern Europeans, and ask why people today have quite different ideas and quite different feelings, you will find that it is because they always had a free etheric component which enabled them to absorb things and transform their nature over the course of time. That is all true in general; but now let us examine in detail how this whole process I have described takes effect.

Imagine that someone were unable to erase from his mind and memory any impression he had received, but retained it. It would be a curious state of affairs if you retained for ever after every impression you received from childhood on, every day of your life from morning to evening. As you know, this all remains present to you for a little while after death, and there is good reason for this. But during life we forget it all. All of you have not only forgotten countless things that you experienced in childhood but also a great deal that happened last year, and no doubt even some of what happened to you yesterday. But a thought that has vanished from your mind, that you have 'forgotten', has by no means vanished entirely from your whole being, from your whole spiritual organism. This is certainly not the case. If you saw a rose yesterday, and have now forgotten it, the picture of the rose remains in you nevertheless, along with the other impressions you absorbed, even if your immediate awareness has forgotten them.

Now there is a very great difference between an idea we have in our mind, and the same idea when it has vanished from memory. So let us consider a thought which we have formed in response to an external impression and which is still present in our mind. And then let us observe, inwardly, how this gradually fades, is gradually forgotten. Yet it is still there, it remains in our whole spiritual organism. What does it do there? What is this apparently forgotten thought preoccupied with in us? It has a very important function. You see, it only properly starts to work upon this free part of the etheric body I have described, and to make this free element of the etheric body useful to us, once it has been forgotten. Only then, in a sense, has it been 'digested'. As long as we use it to know something, it does not work inwardly upon the free mobility, the organization of the free part of the etheric body. The moment it lapses into forgetfulness, it begins to work. And so we can say that work is continually being accomplished in the free part of the human etheric body, work is being done upon it. And what exactly is working there? The forgotten thoughts. That is the great blessing of forgetting. As long as a thought remains in your mind, you keep relating it to an object. When you look at a rose, and have the idea or picture of it in your mind, you are relating the thought of the rose to the external object. The thought is bound up with the outward object and has to send its inner energy towards it. But the moment you forget the thought, it is released and begins to develop germinal powers which work inwardly upon the human etheric body. Our forgotten thoughts are therefore of key importance for us. A plant cannot forget, nor of course can it receive impressions. But it could not forget anyway because it uses its whole etheric body to grow, leaving nothing over. If thoughts could enter the plant, there would be nothing within it that could work upon them and develop them.

Everything that happens does so through lawful necessity. Wherever there is something that needs to develop but finds no support for this development, the latter meets hindrance. Everything in an organism that is not incorporated into development becomes a hindrance to development. Let us imagine that the interior of the eye were to secrete all kinds of particles, substances that could not be assimilated into the general aqueous humour of the eye: our vision would be disturbed. Nothing should remain over that is not inwoven, incorporated, assimilated. The same is true of mental or spiritual impressions. Someone, for instance, who continually retained in his mind the impressions he received could easily arrive at a condition in which the part of him that should be nourished by forgotten thoughts received too little of them, and then this part would disrupt his development like a paralysed limb instead of nurturing it. This also explains why it is harmful for someone to lie awake at night unable to rid his mind of his impressions, of certain anxieties. If he could forget them, they would begin to work wholesomely upon his etheric body. This shows the tangible blessing of forgetting; and here at the same time you can see why it is necessary not to compulsively keep hold of this or that thought, but instead learn to forget certain things. It is very injurious to a person's inner well-being and state of health if he is unable to forget certain things.

These are very ordinary matters of daily life, but they also apply to ethical and moral considerations. Someone who does not hold grudges can be experienced as wholesome and benevolent. Our health is eaten up if we hold grudges. If someone has done us an injury, and we absorb the impression of what he did to us and keep going over it in our mind, keep coming back to it whenever we see him, we relate this thought of injury to the person concerned and allow it to emanate from us. But let us imagine, instead, that we succeed in shaking the hand of the person who harmed us when we meet him again, that we behave as if nothing had happened. In truth, that is wholesome. It is not just metaphorical to say this but a reality: it has a healing and beneficial effect. Such a thought, seemingly dull and ineffective outwardly, at the same moment pours itself into us like healing balm for a great deal we carry within us. These things are realities, and can show us a further aspect of the blessing of forgetting. Forgetting is not simply a deficiency for us but something that belongs to the most beneficial aspects of human life. If we only developed our memory, and if we retained in it everything that makes an impression on us, our etheric body would have to bear more and more, would gain ever richer content and yet at the same time would grow ever more inwardly arid. Our capacity to develop is something we owe to our ability to forget. And yet it is still true to say that no thought completely vanishes from us; and we can see this best in the great panorama of our lives that unfolds immediately after death. There we see that no impression is ever completely lost.

Having touched on the blessing of forgetting in daily life, both in more neutral and in moral domains, we can consider how it works in the great compass of life between death and a new birth. What exactly is the nature of kamaloka, that transitional period before we enter devachan,[10] the world of spirit as such? This kamaloka exists because immediately after death we cannot yet forget the inclinations, desires and pleasures we had in life. At death we first depart from our physical body and then the great memory tableau stands before our soul, as often described. This fades completely after two, three or at the most four days, leaving behind a kind of essence of the etheric body. While the actual, full etheric body draws away from us and dissolves in the general world ether, a kind of framework or shell of the etheric body remains behind, but contracted to an essence. The astral body is the bearer of all instincts, drives, desires, passions, feelings, emotions and pleasures. Now in kamaloka the astral body could not come to awareness of tormenting privation if it did not continually have the opportunity, through its connection with the residues of the etheric body, to recall what it enjoyed and desired in life. And shedding this habit of desires is really nothing other than a gradual forgetting of what chains us to the physical world. In seeking to enter devachan we must first learn to forget what chains us to the physical world. Here we see how we are tormented by still remembering the physical world. Just as cares and anxieties can torment us when we cannot get rid of them from our mind, so our still remaining desires and instincts torment us too after death. And this tormenting memory of our involvement in life expresses itself in everything we must pass through in the period of kamaloka. And only when we have succeeded in forgetting all the desires and wishes we had in relation to the physical world do the achievements and fruits of our life just past emerge in a way that enables them to work as they must in devachan. Here they become shapers and crafters to form our new life. Basically we can say that in devachan we work at the new form we should have when we return to earthly life. This work, this preparation of our subsequent nature, gives us the sense of bliss that we feel throughout the period of devachan. Having passed through kamaloka, we embark on the preparatory work for our future form. Life in devachan is always taken up by using the essence or extract we have received to develop the archetype of our next human form. We develop this archetype by incorporating the fruits of our past life into it. But we can only do this by forgetting the severe hardship we experienced in kamaloka.

The suffering and privation in kamaloka originates in our inability to forget certain connections with the physical world, in the fact that the physical world still hovers before us like a memory. But once we have passed through the 'waters of Lethe', the river of oblivion, and have learned this forgetting, the achievements and experiences of our previous incarnation are used to gradually develop the archetype, the prototype of our next life on earth. And then the bliss and joy of devachan begins to replace suffering. In the same way that in ordinary life, if cares and worries torment us, if certain thoughts refuse to fade from our mind, we are as it were shoving a dead and dried-up stick into our etheric body, so after death we have in us something that goes on contributing to our sufferings and privations for as long as we have not yet swept away all connections with the physical world by forgetting. Just as forgotten ideas and thoughts can become a seed of healing for us, so all experiences of our previous life become a source of joy in devachan once we have crossed the river of forgetfulness, and have forgotten everything that binds us to life in the sense world.

And so we see that these laws of forgetting and remembering also hold true in a broader scope of existence.

Now you might ask this: How can we have any ideas after death about what happened in our previous life if we are obliged to forget this life? You might wonder if the word 'forgetting' is apt at all since we have laid aside our etheric body and yet remembering and forgetting are connected with this etheric body. But after death, of course, remembering and forgetting acquire a different form. Ordinary memory is replaced by reading in the Akashic Records. Whatever happens in the world does not vanish but continues to have an objective existence. As our memory of our connection with physical life fades during kamaloka, these occurrences surface in a quite different way, becoming apparent to us in the Akashic Records. And so we no longer need the connection with our life as ordinary memory provides it. All such questions can be resolved, though we must take the time for this, and gradually deal with them, since it is not possible to immediately explain everything that can make something comprehensible.

Knowing these things that we have been discussing helps explain a great many things in daily life. Much that belongs to the human etheric body can be discerned in the distinctive way the temperaments affect us. We have said that these enduring characteristics, which we call the 'temperaments', have their origin in the etheric body. A person with a melancholic temperament, who cannot leave certain thoughts behind but is compelled to keep revisiting them, is quite different in this respect from someone of a sanguine or phlegmatic temperament whose thoughts keep flitting away.

A melancholic temperament, as we have seen, will be detrimental to a person's health in the sense we have been discussing, whereas a sanguine temperament can to some degree be very beneficial for health. Of course I'm not saying that people should try to forget everything. But you can see from these things why a sanguine or phlegmatic temperament can be healthy, and why a melancholic temperament may not be. The question still remains as to whether a phlegmatic temperament is working in the right way. A phlegmatic who absorbs trivial thoughts will easily forget them, which will indeed be a healthy thing. But if he only has such thoughts, it will not be at all good for him. Various things come into play here.

Spiritual science can answer the question as to whether forgetting is only a deficiency of human nature or perhaps something useful. And from such insight we also see strong moral impulses ensuing. If a person recognizes that it benefits his well-being—in quite objective terms—to be able to forget insults and injuries done to him, a quite different impulse will be present. But as long as he believes that this has no importance, no moral sermons will be of the least use. Once he knows that he should try to forget, and that his well-being depends on it, he will surely let this impulse work in him in a quite different way. We don't have to call this 'egoistic'. We can see it like this: if I am sick and ailing, I am not much use to the world. We can also consider the question of well-being from a quite different perspective. A decided egoist will not find such reflections as these of much use. But someone who cares about the well-being of humanity and is therefore concerned to play his part in this, and so has his own well-being indirectly in view, will be able to draw moral sustenance from such reflections. When spiritual science enters our lives and shows us the truth about certain spiritual circumstances, it will become clear that it can offer us the greatest ethical and moral impulses of a kind provided by no other kind of knowledge, let alone by merely outward moral commandments. Knowledge of the realities of the world of spirit, as communicated by spiritual science, is therefore a strong impulse that can also lead to the greatest progress in the moral life of human beings.

Seminar Discussions on the Temperaments

STUTTGART, AUGUST 1919

Rudolf Steiner draws the following figures on the board:[11]

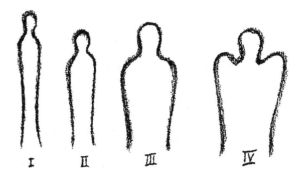

Here we have a characterization of the four temperaments. Melancholic children as a rule are slim and thin. The sanguines appear most normal. Those whose shoulders slope out more are the phlegmatic children. The choleric children are the ones of stocky build, whose head nearly sinks into the body.

In Michelangelo and Beethoven you can see a combination of melancholic and choleric temperament.

Now I'd like you to note that, as teachers, we certainly should not regard the child's temperament as some kind of 'flaw' that needs to be remedied. We should *recognize* the temperament and ask ourselves how to work with it to achieve a desirable goal in life—how to draw the very best out of a particular temperament so that children can use it to achieve their life goals. In the case of the choleric, particularly, it would be of very little use if we tried to extirpate it and replace it with something else. A great deal emerges from the life and passion of the choleric, and much would have been different in world history if cholerics had not existed. In the child, above all we should try to see what goals in life are fitting for him to work towards despite the temperament.

For the choleric, if possible, we should create invented, imagined situations that we present for the child's attention. We can for instance direct the attention of a child in a temper to imagined situations and handle them cholerically ourselves. I might tell a young choleric a story about a wild fellow I met, describing him very vividly. And then I would get in a rage myself and describe how I handle such a fellow, how I view him, so that the choleric child can see choleric nature embodied in someone other than him—in an invented form, so that he can look at such actions. By this means we can draw on the strength in him to enable him to understand other things too.

Temperament extremes

It would be good if you would also consider the extremes of the temperaments. Goethe's world-view enabled him to formulate the lovely thought that the normal can be studied through abnormality.[12] Goethe looks at an abnormal plant, a misshapen plant, and through this malformation he learns about the plant in a normal state. In the same way we can draw lines connecting an entirely normal condition with malformations of body and soul. And you yourselves can find what connects the temperaments to abnormal soul states.

When the melancholic temperament assumes an abnormal, distorted form and, instead of remaining within soul boundaries, encroaches on the body, on corporeal nature, this gives rise to madness. Madness arises, basically, when the melancholic temperament exceeds its due bounds and scope. When the phlegmatic temperament does this, it leads to idiocy. The sanguine temperament degenerates into imbecility, and the choleric into mania. Sometimes, when a person gets very worked up, quite normal states of soul can suddenly change and show signs of madness, idiocy, imbecility or mania. We need to form the habit of observing the whole life of the psyche in this way.

Self-education

Modern culture, especially in its concern with the approaching future of society, will doubtless assign increasing importance to what we can call our self-education. This evening, based on the spiritual-scientific world-view that I propound, I wish to say a few things about this self-education. Given the broad scope of this theme, however, I can only offer certain outlines. Let me first expressly emphasize that I will not be speaking of the kind of self-development that can lead to spiritual research. Instead the subject tonight will be our ordinary, everyday self-education which, in a sense, precedes any further education in spiritual research, and which has importance and value not just for those who pursue the latter but for everyone.

The very word 'self-education' may give many the sense of something contradictory, or at least something whose realization can meet with great obstacles. Why is this? Well, simply because education indicates our approach to something foreign to or beyond us, something that we do not yet possess or master. But self-education naturally means something we ourselves can engage in, where we are therefore both teacher and pupil at once. And this is at the same time a very problematic endeavour.

Let us first summarize what spiritual science says about the education of the child. You can find all this in my little booklet entitled *The Education of the Child in the Light of Spiritual Science*. In this introduction I cannot of course go over everything covered there. But I do want to say that when, in accordance with spiritual science, we consider the real and whole human being and trace his development, we can discover that education up to a certain point of maturation has various primary aims. We find that up to around the age of six, that is, until second dentition, education must start from what we can call the child's capacity for imitation, his urge to imitate. In the booklet I mentioned, what the child sees and hears from adults around him is shown to be more important for his education than all moral rules and any other kind of instruction. Another important stage in the child's life begins with second dentition and lasts roughly until puberty. Here we find, if we shed all preconceptions and examine a person's actual development, that the impulse at work in education during these years must be what we can call authority. Education at this time will be healthy if the child is surrounded by adults in whom he has trust and faith so that, without resorting to some pale rationality or immature criticism, he can form his principles, the rules for his own conduct, under the benign authority of these adults. The principle of authority governs education in this period. The booklet I spoke of explains why this is so. And then, as we follow a person's development further, up to the age of 20 or 21, we find that this development itself, and its underlying conditions, emphasizes the maturing intellect, especially the need to look up to an impersonal ideal encompassed in the soul, and thus to a purely spiritual educational impulse. As yet this exceeds what the young person himself can be at this age. That of course is the very nature of an ideal—something we strive towards, always having a sense, especially in our youth, that our whole conduct and our whole being as yet fall far short. The ideal hovers over us like the dome of the heavens, and we strive for it with an awareness that we can never actually attain it.

Only when this period is past do we really arrive at the point in our life when we can embark on our self-education, or when we can speak of self-education in the narrower sense. Apart from the third and last educational impulse—although this too is such that a young person draws here on ideals from the great movements of world history or elsewhere, and in other words seeks them outside himself—the others, such as the principle of authority, are founded on an ideal relationship with someone outside him, someone, therefore, who is assumed to be more advanced or perfect than he is. Thus the pupil sees the impulses which his education brings him as something outside himself. He looks up to them.

When we come to speak of self-education as such, it is quite natural that we can no longer discuss it in the same terms as we do the educational impulses for earlier years. There is a contrast and contradiction here—not a merely logical one but more philosophical. If we are to become our own teacher, we have to assume that the impulses for this already lie within us. If we are to educate ourselves, isn't it really highly likely that instead of broadening our horizons and perfecting ourselves, or enriching our lives, we actually constrict them? Is it not likely that we undertake a self-education according to ideas we already possess, that we already have a mind to pursue or that we have already absorbed, and that in fact we undermine the rich possibilities that are seeking to emerge from within us and easily narrow our horizons through self-education rather than broadening and perfecting them? Isn't this contradiction highly possible?

The nature of our culture today means that ever greater emphasis is, necessarily, placed on self-education, on education, on the individual person. We can understand this. There is no need to look back to ancient India or trace its legacy in the modern world, nor to ancient Egypt, to see, in both cases, how a certain caste division placed people into a particular social position from the outset. This made it impossible for them to develop freely, laid down how they should behave in accordance with their position in the social order—and still does so today. We do not have to look back to ancient times to see this, for until quite recently—with effects that very much continue to reverberate—people's lives were determined by, say, blood relationships, class and caste divisions and so on. At the same time we also see how something quite different is emerging from this social fabric, something that increasingly places people in direct connection with each other, so that they meet face to face as it were in the social order. And beside this more direct encounter between people we also see how each person has to be increasingly self-reliant in relation to nature and the whole universe. We see how each person becomes reliant on his own view and judgement as life goes on, on the convictions forming in his soul, on the way in which he conceives of, and reflects on, moral, aesthetic and religious matters. And it is quite self-evident that a person thrown back upon himself must try to discover in the depths of his soul what connects

Right opinion

him as one human being with others and what, in general, places him in a satisfying position in relation to the rest of the world.

In this context it is understandable that there is, inevitably, an increasing clamour for self-education. How people should behave in life in accordance with specific, traditional rules can be taught to children as part of their education. But this will not suffice as our lives inevitably change and develop. The conditions at work in such development cannot be suppressed by any power in the world. It becomes apparent that we must repeatedly feel the call, in every situation, to keep an open mind and develop an unprejudiced perspective whenever we meet another person. Throughout our lives we must work upon ourselves to develop ever greater perfection in our whole outlook on the world. The most important impulses for such conduct are not actually given us in childhood but rather when we strive to find our own place in the world. When, at the right age, we become self-reliant, and can no longer seek submission to other educators, we have to become our own guide and teacher—in other words, become the one who makes us ever better and more perfect as human beings. Thus everywhere in literature and public life we can today witness a flood of reflections and observations on personal development, on endeavours to live more harmoniously and so on. This is entirely understandable in our day and age, even self-evident. But anyone who can see deeper into things will soon notice that these contemporary efforts at self-improvement just described are more likely to lead to a curtailing of life, a narrowing of its horizons, than to its perfection and enrichment.

Right judgement

Here we see authors wedded to the ideal of helping people by instructing them in ways to work upon their life of thought. Some will tend more towards physical measures, recommending things that they themselves may perhaps most favour, based on their personal taste and personal sympathies: giving all kinds of external bodily exercises, or recommending a particular diet, or a way of dividing up the day and suchlike. As I said, such principles are propounded all over the place today, in life and literature. This does not mean that we should automatically reject such endeavours. There may be a great deal that is good in them. Yet many such things act in only a one-sided way, such as recommendations based on the book *In Tune with the Infinite* by Ralph Waldo Trine.[13] You see, it has to be said that someone who devotes himself to such efforts and forms a narrowly circumscribed idea of how to develop harmony in life will not really develop, enrich or perfect his life forces, but rather constrain, confine and limit them. This is so even if these very limitations perhaps lead to a momentary sense of well-being or inner satisfaction or even feelings of bliss. Here it is easy to overlook the fact that such efforts in modern times can give rise to the most curious or far-fetched oddities, allowing each person, without much thought or study, to praise as universally human things that he simply inclines to personally. It is necessary to look deeper into human nature if we are to speak of self-education as spiritual science understands it. The distinctive nature of spiritual science is that it avoids the one-sided limitations of other endeavours, which it finds to be small circles encompassed within its greater circumference. Through dedication to the whole of human nature, it seeks to perceive conditions affecting each separate human life. It is always easier to pursue a particular bias that promises, say, that you will quickly regain your health or improve your memory or achieve practical success in life. The path of spiritual science is less easy, asks more of us; but it is a path founded on the whole nature and essence of the human being.

Now when we speak of self-education, we may perhaps gather how best to pursue it by understanding that at an age when our youth makes it necessary for others to educate us a certain degree of self-education already comes into play. This might seem a still bigger contradiction than the one I mentioned earlier, but in fact it is not. Spiritual science, you see, shows us that the human self is something more extensive than it appears within the confines of our immediate personality. Actually, the whole spiritual-scientific outlook is based on the fact that we can to some degree get beyond ourselves, beyond what is enclosed within the confines of our personality, but without losing ourselves in the process. Is there any example in ordinary life of what spiritual science seeks to embody in a much more comprehensive way in all areas of life? Yes. There are two things in daily life which already show that we can get beyond our personal concerns and yet, as it were, remain with ourselves, not lose ourselves. One of these is human sympathy, compassion, shared joy— what we call compassionate love. What gives rise to this love, this sympathy, this sharing of others' pleasure? These qualities do not appear so very mysterious to us only because we easily accept what we are used to. Just as native people may not ask *why* the sun rises and sets but simply accept it, and only begin to reflect on what causes this as culture develops, so in ordinary life we do not give much thought to sympathy and sharing in another's feelings. Only as we start to seek illumination about life's purpose and meaning does human sympathy and compassion become more enigmatic, something veiled in mystery. We need only think of one thing alone and we will quickly see that sympathy and sharing another's joy are an enlargement of the human self as it first presents itself.

Joy and suffering, as we experience them individually, are the most intimate and inward of experiences. If we look at someone else and an impulse arises within us that mirrors in us his suffering or joy, then we are no longer merely living within ourselves but also in the other. And all philosophical speculation that, say, something is triggered in us here by a sense impression cannot deceive us to the reality: that when we share in another's joys and sufferings something is actively at work within us. When we intimately feel the other's joy or suffering, we have emerged from ourselves and have entered the inner sanctum of the other person, have entered what we feel, within ourselves, to be our most essential being. And since, as no one will deny, we cannot transport our mind into the other person's mind, we need only think this: that if at the moment we shared the feeling of a soul distinct and separate from us we were to experience ourselves within this other soul in a kind of helpless, powerless state, then it would not be possible to enter into another person without at the same time losing ourselves. As strange as this sounds, it is very important for life: we enter into another being, and yet no sense of impotence overwhelms us. We emerge from our-

Right action

selves and live within the other, yet we do not succumb or grow faint as we do so.

All spiritual-scientific development unfolds in precise accordance with this model, and in no other way. Just as we can enter into another person without losing ourselves when we share in his suffering or pleasure, so in spiritual research it is possible to enter into other entities without loss of self. This isn't possible in ordinary life, since when we ordinarily depart from ourselves on a quest to know and perceive we fall asleep—we are no longer with or within ourselves. In ordinary life we do not do what we achieve in moral life in the single instance of sympathy and compassion. This distinctive quality of shared feeling is therefore the model for all spiritual-scientific activity, which unfolds in the same way sympathy and compassion unfold in normal circumstances. Here is one instance where we can get beyond our own individuality without losing ourselves.

The other, likewise in the realm of morality in ordinary life, is what we experience as the impulse of conscience. If we study the workings of conscience—we have spoken about this here before—we know that when we hear the voice of conscience we hear something that reaches beyond our personal sympathies and antipathies, and indeed can even act as a powerful corrective to them. And again it is true that in the moral domain, when this voice of conscience leads us beyond ourselves, we do not lose ourselves or succumb to helplessness. All spiritual science depends upon our ability to enter a sphere that lies outside our person, a realm which our everyday consciousness can encompass but within which we do not lose ourselves as we move within it. Indeed, if we look at this with an open mind, surely we can say that on this depends also our insight into repeated lives on earth, frequently discussed in these lecture series, and our understanding of causes and effects passing from one life to the next. This insight also depends on the same capacity. Viewing our life between birth and death with ordinary awareness, we can learn through spiritual science to see that this scope of existence, which we judge, and lodge in memory, can be regarded as our personal self. But we also learn to see that we can, in thought, depart from this personal self and rise to a self that now does not live only through the instrument of our body but rather works to develop this body. We can come to see that this too is the self, not only living in a body between birth and death but passing through many births and deaths and repeatedly appearing on earth. Even though people ordinarily have no memory of former stages of their life on earth and can only gain a theoretical conviction of the truth of repeated earthly lives and of the effects of causes that work through from one human incarnation into another, nevertheless they can postulate that what exists in us is not limited to our person as it appears here, that what lives in us is in a sense transpersonal—it creates our present self and appears within it as active principle. In the same way that we have a direct experience of going beyond ourselves in our conscience, in our sharing of others' feelings, so spiritual-scientific research can experience entry into a higher realm. Yet if we fully understand spiritual science, we will never admit that we lose ourselves in this higher realm. Here, rather, something holds sway with which we are connected, to which we belong, and in which we truly do not lose ourselves, despite doing so initially with our ordinary everyday awareness.

Thus the science of the spirit is modelled on our encompassing of a higher self when we share others' feelings of joy and sorrow without losing ourselves. And so when we become aware of our enlarged self, through which we enter into the experience of other beings, we can consider the child and see that he not only develops through normal states of consciousness that we have foremost in mind as teachers, but that apart from his ordinary self a higher being outside it is working upon the child. If we consider this, we may find something in the child in which a kind of education is at work, whereas with our ordinary educational measures we can only address the child's personal self. Where do we find this higher self active as a higher entity belonging to the child but not entering his awareness? It may sound strange but we find this active in the child in absorbed, focused play. In the child at play we can only create the context, the conditions for education to happen. What is achieved through play is basically achieved through the child's own activity, through all that we cannot harness within strict rules. That is the key thing about play, its educational value: that our rules cease here, our pedagogical and educational arts, and we leave the child to his own powers. What does the child do when we leave him to his own resources? In play he uses outer objects to see if something works through his own activity. He activates his own will, brings it into movement. And through the way in which external things behave in response to his will, the child educates himself quite differently from an education undertaken by another person or in line with his pedagogical principles. He educates himself directly through life, albeit only playfully. This is why it is so important that we refrain as far as possible from bringing logic and intellect to bear upon the child's play. The more play unfolds in a non-conceptual way, in what is perceived in a living element, the better it will be. If we give a child toy figures, human or animal, with strings or threads that can be pulled to create the appearance of movement, whether this be in a picture book or otherwise, it will allow him a better education through play than if we give him the finest building blocks. There is already too much rationality involved in the latter, and this belongs to a more personal principle than to a living, mobile engagement with things not conceptually understood but instead encompassed in their holistic activity. The less pre-determined and conceptually designed play is, the better it will be. And this is because a higher element cannot be forced into human awareness, but only enters as the child tries out and tests things in a living context, non-intellectually. Here we see how the child can be educated by something that goes beyond the personal realm.

In a sense, play remains an important educational factor throughout life. Naturally I don't mean playing cards or suchlike, for all games that employ reason, combinative thinking, draw on the personal element in us, which is most bound up with the instrument of the brain. However bene-ficial chess may be in some respects, it can never become part of self-education because it draws on what is most bound up with the instrument of the brain, on what must create com-binations. When we engage in gymnastic play on the other hand, in gymnastic exercises, and must set our muscles in motion without use of combinative reason but instead by learning directly from the muscles, and thus from activity rather than comprehension, such play is self-educative. We here discover a principle that is important in all self-education: that when we try to educate ourselves both through education of the will and of the intellect, the education of the will first and foremost, this will education, this culture of the will, depends on our cultivating an engagement with the outer world and a reciprocal relationship with it. The human will cannot be educated by training inner thought processes. It is strengthened, rather, so that we gain a stable inner point of support in ourselves, when we seek this culture of the will in a reciprocal relationship between our own will and the outer world. This is why it is harmful to a considerable degree for ordinary, outer, daily self-education if we try to strengthen our will for outward life by means of inner training measures and methods.

Here we come to various things that are widely recommended measures of self-education today but which a truly spiritual-scientific perspective must warn against in no uncertain terms. People are advised how they can make a self-confident impression on others, how they can train their will so that they can engage in life and act in a way that corresponds to their intentions. For instance they are told to undertake exercises to overcome fear, or curiosity, or other passionate or negative feelings. In other words, they are urged to work upon their negative feelings and emotions. I know that many who now hear me say this will later think I am opposed to mastering fear, passions and so on. But that is not so. What I am saying, rather, is that demands of this kind that a person makes upon himself cannot lead to any real, useful will culture in outward life. You see, this culture of the will, which we need for outward life, is something we must acquire through reciprocal relationship and engagement with it. When someone needs a strong will for life it is a much better thing to try to acquire this by trying and proving his outer strength, exerting his body and attending with his eyes, and thus really taking up battle with the immediate sense world around him. This is what brings us into true harmony with the external world—the same world through which the play of our muscles and our whole physical organization has been formed, though formed of course out of the spiritual realm.

But by guiding our self-education in this way, we are also working on the parts of our spiritual organism that lead us to harmony with the outer world immediately surrounding us. If we work only inwardly, with mental exercises and so forth, as these figure in popular books today, we are working at one remove from the world, in this constrained and limited soul which is not in harmony with the world but whose significance consists in the very fact that it separates itself from it. It is true to say, therefore, that someone who exposes himself to outward dangers and tries to overcome them is practising a better form of self-education than another who goes and buys books on self-development and starts doing exercises to overcome fear, emotions and so on. While these relatively easy things may lead to all kinds of personal advantages, this is always at the cost of developing something that isolates him from the world, whereas what I first described will place him selflessly into it. As I said, some may therefore say that I am opposed to overcoming fear and other emotions, to everything in fact that might be thought to belong to self-education. But it is only in one instance that I emphasize this: when it is a matter of developing our will for outer, physical life, when we are trying to strengthen the will in outward life, and this is because inner exercises are misplaced when it is a matter of character development, of will education. They are rightly applied, on the other hand, to educating our knowledge and perceptions.

Those who wish to achieve knowledge and insight, who wish to penetrate the supersensible world, and have no aim, to begin with, other than seeing into the supersensible world, will be right to do such exercises. And this is why spiritual science is quite precise and specific in *not* asking, 'How do we gain forces to develop the will in daily life?' but instead, 'How do we gain knowledge of the higher worlds?' The terms used here are very precise. In fact, as these things are described in my book *Knowledge of the Higher Worlds*, they do also lead to a culture of the will—not directly but indirectly. You see, someone who seeks to develop faculties of perception of the higher worlds must await what then comes towards him. The development of the will must arise by itself, and then it acts rightly and takes healthy paths.

And so we can say that cultivating the will, educating the will, must initially be based on a person developing a healthy relationship especially between his physical nature in the world and that external world, whether he does this more by cultivating bodily abilities or when he seeks something relating more to character development. Here, rather than brooding on how one can become fearless and overcome certain emotions, it will be much more important to face what life presents us with, what happens between us and others, and then to give ourselves up to unselfconscious feelings, the play of marked nuances of feeling that tend either more towards sympathy or antipathy. By taking our path through life in this way, cultivating our participation in life in all circumstances, with all its nuances, we make ourselves into a place of interplay with the outer world that can really lead our will onwards by successive stages. It schools our will to engage with life fully, with all the sympathies and antipathies this elicits from us. In other words, what leads us beyond ourselves into the world develops our will. And everything that leads us away from the world, that leads us deeper into ourselves, schools our knowledge and perception, and in this case does so on the right basis. When we seek to develop our own knowledge and independent existence this helps the progress of our inner life. Our own insights and knowledge, it must be said, lie in the realm of our personal inner development. By developing our powers of cognition and perception, acquiring inner powers, we become more harmonious in our outlook on life, and in our capacity to grasp life's riddles. By contrast, in the context of ordinary everyday life the will is schooled only by engaging with life itself.

This can at the same time tell us where we should seek the teacher who, in the case of self-education, is we ourselves. Except that this teacher must not be our own narrower self, particularly not when it comes to educating our own will. When spiritual science enables us to take wing and go beyond the bounds of our own personality without, however, losing

ourselves, then, as we engage directly in life itself and allow
life to work upon us, we educate ourselves, our will—and
please don't misunderstand the comparison—in the same
way that play works upon the child. But how does this happen? Well, there is a way of understanding and viewing life by
trying to inform everything with our reason. This culture of
rationality does not in fact help us progress, and therefore has
no value in our self-education. The greatest role in our self-
education is played by what reaches beyond intellectualism
and reason as we acquire maturity. Just as a child is best
educated by playing, by trying things out, rather than intellectual instruction, so a person will best educate his will
through experiences in life that he does not comprehend
logically, but towards which he feels a connection of sympathy, of love, a sense of the sublimity or humour of things.
This helps us progress. Here lies the self-education of our
will. Reason and intellectual culture usually cannot work
upon the will at all. But now let us study how direct experiences act upon the will.

A moral philosopher, Carneri, who does not embrace the
point of view of reincarnation, points out that a child's
character is constant yet developing, and forms precisely
through elements that arise directly from life. Then he asks
this: What can make a person's character change in only a
brief period? He says that someone can change radically, for
example, through a powerful love or through a friendship in
which a person suddenly feels uncritical sympathy for
another; he loses himself in the other. And then his character
can suddenly take a quite different turn simply because in the
spheres where character is rooted, that is, where the will is

active, our sensibility and emotions play directly into life. When we meet another and perceive him to be an excellent or bad person, using our reason in this judgement, our character does not change, for otherwise judges would change many times a week. But when feelings of friendship and affinity arise, a person's whole configuration of character can often alter. This is firm proof that cultivating our will depends on developing our sensibility and feelings in relation to and through life itself. But since we can to some degree take our life in hand and effect a certain correction of our feelings and outlook, we also have the capacity to educate our will to some extent. But here it is a matter of attending to life, not simply living regardless and giving ourselves up easily to the flow of life, but attending, paying attention. And so we see that we can better educate ourselves if we succeed in getting some grip on our feelings and moods, and that someone who never masters his feelings and moods but continually loses himself in them will be the worst self-educator.

If we seek, therefore, to educate our own will, we must address our feelings and emotions if this is to be directly achieved. We must enquire in wise self-knowledge how we can work upon our feelings and emotions. The moment to do this, however, is not when we lose ourselves in sympathy or antipathy. We therefore have to choose carefully the moments when we educate our will, at times when we are not particularly taken up with our moods and feelings: when we are able to reflect on our life and our emotions. This means that self-education must be practised at the moments when least is required of us in this way. And yet that is when people do it least, since they are unruffled at such times. Only when we succumb again to our moods and feelings may we notice that we failed to do such work. And later, when free to some degree of involvement in life, we forget to do it—it seems of no concern. This is one of the most important laws, that we must educate the will in and through life by wisely taking in hand the way our feelings unfold.

By contrast, the will is always developed in an egoistic, self-seeking direction if we base this will training on intellectual culture, using the intellect to strengthen and empower the will. Such exercises are directly relevant to our knowledge culture, for what we seek to achieve in the realm of the mind and later even of the soul. Here, though, we can do nothing other than work on ourselves within our soul. It is of very great importance in this case for us to weigh up a great contradiction existing between the self-cultivation of inner or of outward life. Error upon error is made in relation to both the first and the second—endless one-sided measures. All kinds of physical measures are recommended for the human body. It may have grown less popular now but there are still people today who wrap themselves up completely and even say that this protects them against excessive heat. More common nowadays is to recommend the one-sided approach of 'toughening people up': rather than protecting themselves against cold and the vagaries of weather, they try to expose themselves to sun and air, believing in the benefits of this. Whether someone exposes himself to the heat of the sun or not, for reasons that he is usually very vague about—in some circumstances this can be very beneficial, though not necessarily part of self-education—or takes endless coldwater cures is not the important thing. The key thing for the body, to put it in a nutshell, is diversity and variation: exposing it to cold sometimes without catching cold, or sometimes walking across a square in the hot, unshaded midday sun. We can therefore say that wise self-education usually cannot be based on most of what is recommended today, but that instead we should try to develop a little of everything to ensure a harmonious effect upon us.

The very opposite of what is good for our body benefits the spirit and the soul. Whereas the outward body needs diversity and adaptation to outward conditions, the soul needs to cultivate the intellect through concentration by repeatedly leading the sum of thoughts, emotions and perceptions back to a few basic ideas. Someone who does not strive to do this as part of his self-education—to reduce the scope of his knowledge to a few fundamentals that can be sovereign over everything else—will see his memory start to suffer in consequence, likewise his nervous system, and the way in which he engages with life. Those who succeed in encapsulating certain things in ruling ideas will find, when outward life requires them to act, that they face it with great equanimity. But those who instead pass through life without doing this, without subsuming what life presents under a few over-arching ideas, will see, firstly, that they find it harder to remember, that they become less fruitfully engaged in life, but also that they bring a certain disharmony to bear on life. And since there is so little faith today in concentrating the mind, and this is so little undertaken in consequence, a great many other ills arise too, and manifest as deficiencies in self-education—above all, what is usually called nervousness.

Whereas we school the will by allowing out muscles their interplay with external life, their interaction with it, we must school our nervous system by concentrating the mind. In other words, everything that works from within outwards and eventually manifests in the nervous system is cultivated and supported by memory and mindfulness, by summing up life in certain ideas. Nurturing the nervous system and the mind and spirit underlying it is necessary if a person is to meet life with inner stability.

When we discuss these questions, a modern, materialistic view easily imposes itself although, from the perspective of moden humanity, there is also much to be disputed in an older outlook. Here people usually confuse two things. A person does not become nervous through the schooling of his will but through its mistaken schooling. Cultivation of the will can lead to nervousness if we seek it in a mistaken way: if, instead of connecting with the external world and steeling the will through its hindrances and obstacles, we try to use all kinds of inner means that are only effective in our thinking life. In this way our will can easily become nervous. It is thought today that we should treat such nervousness very leniently and forgivingly. Carneri[14] relates an interesting case. An estate owner was a very good-natured man yet sometimes he fell into such a state that he started to beat his servants. This was thought to be a special case of nervousness and the man was pitied for it. The estate owner's servants suffered a great deal from his mood swings, but modern experts expressed infinite regret that the poor man must live with such a condition, repeatedly beating his servants in this way. As Carneri himself relates, this came to a head one day when the man he was about to wrongfully punish himself picked up a stick and beat the landowner so that the latter had to take to his bed for a week. What happened was this: whereas people were previously wont to pity the landowner for his moods, they now stopped doing so; and after a while he seemed completely changed. I am not recommending any course of action here myself, but such a reality of life is really very instructive. If we take a closer look it is easy to see that just speaking to the landowner would not have affected his nervousness. Acting only on his reason and intellect, no reciprocal interplay with the outer world would have come about, and he would have remained unchanged. But he did interact with it, or rather the other man's stick interacted with him. In the former case he would never have learned something which he did learn as he actually met life: in the fullest sense he met the effect arising from his state of soul, his nervousness. We must therefore correct our idea of will schooling so that we understand that the will can only be cultivated when it steels itself in contact with the outer world, albeit not always of course in such a drastic way as the story I told you relates.

As far as the mental life is concerned in self-education, we need to be able to live inwardly in a way that awakens the element that renders us inwardly fruitful. This lies within us, but can lie fallow, can remain arid. We develop it by gathering up our store of perceptions, repeatedly perusing them, looking back at certain ideas and surveying our experiences, continually examining what is there. In particular it is very important that we do not only cultivate reason, that we not only remember, think and picture but, much more important and essential, learn to forget in the right way. This is part of healthy self-education. I'm not recommending forgetting here as a special virtue. It is like this: when we have a certain experience in life, we quickly notice that we cannot carry its full scope with us into a later moment. We can sometimes do this with thoughts, but only very rarely with emotions, feelings, pain and sufferings. But how do these work on in us? They fade away, and work on in the hidden depths of our soul life. What is forgotten becomes a healthy element sinking into these hidden depths. And by sinking down in us in this way, this healthy element becomes something that works upon us, that can help us progress from stage to stage. It is not a matter of stuffing ourselves full, as it were, with all kinds of material but rather of attentively observing things, retaining what we need while the rest of our experience sinks down into the soul's depths. Here we cultivate our intellectual element, nurture the element of attention which is especially important. Anyone who does not think this especially important will not take himself, his own personality in hand. But if we know that what we forget is important then we recognize that we should take our own life in hand and not just let everything act upon us. If I am in a group of gossiping people where not much of interest is being said, I may very well forget it; but what matters is whether I forget this unintelligent gossip or something healthy, more wise or judicious. You see, it matters *what* we forget, what we include in our forgetting. From what we forget, something often surfaces which will now be the subject of our creative imagination. Whereas reason is an element that tires and exhausts life, everything that brings our soul faculties into motion so that we can invent and create is a fruitful, enlivening and life-enhancing element. This is something we must particularly cultivate in well-governed self-education.

We have considered a few aspects of self-education in relation to the intellect and the inner element of soul; and if we especially cultivate this inner soul element, placing chief emphasis upon it, we will see that it also flows entirely by itself into our will, into our character. By contrast, all our efforts to directly influence our character are more likely to weaken it since then we are not engaging in a reciprocal relationship with the whole world.

Spiritual science can teach us about the law of repeating lives on earth, and the law of karma—that is, that what I experience in this life results from former lives, and will in turn give rise to what I encounter and experience in future lives. This supports and sustains everything that can serve our self-education. If we integrate into our lives ideas about reincarnation and karma, we can learn to establish the right alternation between acceptance or acquiescence and self-instigated activity. In relation to these two qualities we can commit the gravest errors. Nowadays people actually handle these two things—acceptance and activity—in the very opposite of a beneficial way for wise self-education. Someone who acknowledges reincarnation will recognize that his destiny in this life, the pain and joy that connects him with one person or another, say, must be understood as governed and caused by himself, the self above and beyond his narrower personality. Then we arrive at something that might at first seem like a weakness: surrendering to our destiny, an

acceptance of our destiny because we know that we ourselves
have tailored it. Things must happen to us as they do because
they have become as they are through our agency. This kind
of surrender to our destiny will strengthen and intensify our
will because it comes about through our relationship to our
outward destiny rather than by will training as such. There is
nothing that can better strengthen our will than surrender to,
and acceptance of, destiny. We can call this composure. You
weaken your will if you grumble at every opportunity and get
indignant about how life treats you. You strengthen your will
by surrendering to your destiny: this is wise self-education.
The people with the weakest will are those who feel that
whatever happens is entirely undeserved and they must
simply shake it off.

Such surrender is often something to which modern
people are averse. Instead they develop another form of
surrender all the more so. Today there is widespread surrender to what exists within us, our reason and inner faculties. People immediately surrender to their inner state of soul
and think that if they do not much like what they find within
them that is their own fault, that they have not paid good
enough attention. Those who get most indignant about their
outward destiny in life surrender most willingly to their inner
state. In this regard people are really very self-satisfied—
especially when they keep reiterating that what already lies
within them is all that they need to develop and pursue.
Modern doctrines of individuality are really the purest submission. But that this individuality must be led to greater
heights and that one should let no opportunity go by to
further this aim is something in complete conflict with the

sense of inner submission and surrender displayed by modern men of action.

To create harmony between inner humility and activity we need the right alternation between them, and this can only be achieved by attentively and openly observing what life offers us. To keep our interest and attention open is something essential in self-education. As we look towards the future, we can recognize that we are now developing, maturing and unfolding faculties, and these will in future work upon our existence and enrich our destiny. If we extend our view of life beyond this present incarnation and consider what effect may emerge from our present existence, our urge to activity will awaken. We will raise ourselves above our present nature. And our sense of surrender will be rightly activated when we see that what happens to us at present was tailored, created by ourselves.

Thus ideas about reincarnation and karma can fill our destiny with exactly what we need in the modern world. The questions about self-education that are so numerous and insistent today will not find the right answer until spiritual science can be incorporated into the inmost impulse, the inner yearning of truly questing modern souls. Spiritual science is not a campaigning movement but it does want to empower modern people to find and nurture the inmost prompting of their souls. It has always been the case that truth, in different forms appropriate to each age, should serve that age, which at the same time has always rejected it. Spiritual science, too, although it offers the surest foundation for all cultural issues of today and the near future, will not escape the fate of being misunderstood and rejected, and finding itself at odds with the prevailing fashions of the day so that people call it empty fantasy and reverie, if not much worse. But it is precisely when we consider such incisive questions that we see the significance and scope of what spiritual science can and does give us. It is an elixir of life. Despite all opposition to, and mockery of, spiritual science, we can also intimate what it is and what it may become as an elixir of life. In relation to it we—those who recognize its true depths and importance—can think of a phrase that can help raise it above all opposition and misunderstanding. The phrase originates with someone with whom we cannot otherwise always agree but who here hit the nail on the head. Arthur Schopenhauer[15] coined words that accord with the destiny of the truth of spiritual science, which must come to inform all cultural questions today and in the near future. In every century, he says, poor truth has blushed at its paradoxical nature, and yet this is not its fault. She simply cannot assume the enthroned form of universal error. She looks up, sighing, to her protective divinity, Time, who promises her victory and fame, but whose wingbeats are so great and slow that the individual dies before her era dawns.

Modern spiritual science can add here what Schopenhauer was not yet able to. Though the protective divinity, Time, has such great, broad wingbeats that an individual cannot glimpse the truth of the times, and must die before truth is victorious, the science of the spirit can show us that an eternal core lives in this individual, a core being who continually returns and is not limited to the single personality but passes on from life to life.

We can therefore say that even if the wingbeats of Time are

so great and broad that the individual dies away and does not witness truth's victory, nevertheless what lives in us, our self, can, when we depart and emerge from this personality, experience this victory, and all such victories, for new life will always vanquish old death. In its deep foundations of truth, spiritual science will affirm what Lessing[16] said as he took full cognizance of this victory of truth. His words are a shining extract, an essence of all the wisdom of past centuries. What the spiritual enquirer can say about the whole scope of human nature as he looks upon what he can achieve above and beyond his personality, but without losing himself in the process, can be expressed as follows by the soul as the deepest, most significant power of its life: 'Is not all eternity mine?'

For the Days of the Week[17]

It is necessary to pay close, careful attention to certain soul processes which we normally undertake without care or attention. There are eight such processes.

Naturally it is best to undertake *only one* such exercise at a time, for a week or a fortnight for instance, and then add the second and so on; and then start all over again. Exercise eight is in the meantime best done daily. Gradually we achieve real self-knowledge by this means, and can also see what progress we have made. Later—starting with Saturday—one exercise can perhaps be done each day alongside the eighth, lasting for about five minutes, so that a particular exercise always falls on the same day, i.e. the thought exercise on Saturday, resolves on Sunday, speech on Monday, action on Tuesday, composure on Wednesday, and so on.

Saturday

Attend to your *thoughts*. Think only significant thoughts. Gradually learn to distinguish the essential and inessential in your thoughts, the eternal from the transitory, the truth from mere opinion.

When listening to what others say, try to become very still within, and to refrain from all agreement, but especially all dismissive judgement (criticism, rejection) in both thoughts and feelings.

This is known as *right opinion.*

Sunday

Resolve to do something, even the least significant thing, only after full and thoughtful consideration. Try to keep at arm's length all thoughtless action, all meaningless activity. We should always have well-considered reasons for everything. And we should certainly omit to do anything which no significant reason prompts us to.

Once we are convinced that a resolve is right, we should adhere to it in inner constancy.

This is called *right judgement*. It remains independent of sympathy and antipathy.

Monday

Speech. Someone who seeks higher development should only let fall from his lips words that have meaning and purpose. All talking for the sake of it—to pass the time, say—is injurious in this sense.

The normal kind of conversation, where people talk fifteen to the dozen about anything and everything, should be avoided. But this does not mean you should shut yourself off from communication with those around you. In everyday conversation speech should gradually work its way through to meaningfulness. Speak and reply to all, but do so thoughtfully, carefully considering what you say. Never speak without reason! Allow yourself to fall silent. Try not to speak either too little or too much. First listen calmly and then assimilate what you have heard.

This exercise is also called *right speech*.

Tuesday

Outward actions. These should not disturb those around us. When our inner prompting (conscience) leads us to act, we should carefully weigh up how we can best do so for the good of the whole, for the enduring felicity of our fellow human beings, and in accordance with eternal values.

Whenever we act—out of our own initiative—we should very thoroughly weigh up what will result from the way we act.

This is also called *right action.*

Wednesday

Living harmoniously, in accord with both nature and spirit. Do not lose yourself in external things. Avoid everything that brings restlessness and haste into your life.

Try not to rush, nor to be lethargic either. Regard life as a means to work, to develop, and act accordingly.

This is also called *right perspective.*

Thursday

Human striving. Make sure you do nothing that is beyond your powers, nor omit to do anything that lies within them.

Look beyond what happens each day and each moment and set yourself goals (ideals) connected with the highest duties of a human being. For instance, try to develop as suggested in these exercises so that you can later offer all the more help and counsel to those around you, even if this is not yet possible in the immediate future.

We can also summarize this as *letting all previous exercises become habitual.*

Friday

The endeavour to *learn from life* as much as possible.

Nothing occurs that does not give us cause to gather experiences that are useful for life. If we have done something wrong or imperfectly, this can cause us to do something similar in a right or more perfect way in future.

When we see others act we can observe them with a similar aim in mind (but not unlovingly). And we do nothing without looking back to experiences that can help us in our decisions and undertakings.

If we are attentive we can learn a great deal from every person, also from children.

This exercise is also called *right memory*—that is, remembering what has been learned from experiences we have had.

In summary

From time to time, look inwards, even if only for five minutes each day at the same time. Entering into contemplation, we should carefully examine and shape the guiding principles of our life, going over in our mind our insights (or lack of them), weighing up our tasks, reflecting on the content and true purpose of life, and feeling serious displeasure at our own mistakes and imperfections. In a word, we should try to distinguish what is essential and enduring, and earnestly set ourselves appropriate goals, for instance virtues that we need to develop. (Never succumb to the error of thinking we have done something well, but instead always strive to emulate the highest exemplars.)

This exercise is also called *right contemplation.*

Notes

Introduction

1. GA 310, Arnheim 24 July 1924, p. 165 (all page nos. refer to German editions).
2. GA 301, Basel, 11 May 1920, p. 231.
3. See Peter Sloterdijk, *Du musst dein Leben ändern* (2009).
4. Marco Bischof, *Salutogenese—unterwegs zur Gesundheit* (2010).
5. Further comments and explanations relating to the temperaments can be found in Rudolf Steiner, *The Four Temperaments*, Rudolf Steiner Press, 2008.
6. For more on this see articles by Harald Haas in *Merkurstab*: Haas, H. (2006), 'Das Verständnis der Aufmerksamkeits-Defizit-Störung auf der Grundlage des Nevositätsbegriffs bei Rudolf Steiner'; in: *Der Merkurstab* 59 (2), pp. 131–42; and Haas, H. (2007), 'Nervosität, die Entwicklung des Seelischen und die heilpädagogischen Konstitutionen', in *Der Merkurstab* 60 (3), pp. 196–207.
7. Rudolf Steiner, *Reinkarnation und Karma* (Rudolf Steiner Verlag 2008).
8. See GA 130, Leipzig 4 and 5 November 1911; GA 134, Hanover, 27 and 28 December 1911; GA 143, Cologne, 8 May 1912.

Forgetting

9. See the chapter 'Gedächtnis' in the work—contained in Rudolf Steiner's library—by Gustav Eichhorn: *Vererbung, Gedächtnis und transzendentale Erinnerung vom Standpunkte des Physikers*, Stuttgart 1909, pp. 41–63; and, also mentioned

elsewhere by Steiner, the book by Gustav Theodor Fechner, *Nanna oder über das Seelenleben der Pflanzen*, 4th edition, Hamburg and Leipzig 1908.

10. Devachan is an Indian expression for the supersensible realm which is called 'heaven' in Christian terminology.

Seminar Discussions on the Temperaments

Second seminar discussion, Stuttgart, 22 August 1919, GA 295, pp. 27–9 and 46f.

11. Unfortunately these original drawings were not preserved. The illustration used here is based on a copy made at the time.

12. See *Die Metamorphose der Pflanze*, § 7 (pp. 20–21) and *Verfolg/ Nacharbeiten und Sammlungen* (pp. 147ff) in Volume 1 of *Goethes Naturwissenschaftliche Schriften*, edited with a commentary by Rudolf Steiner in *Kürschners Deutsche National-Litteratur* (1883/ 97) (GA 1a–e), reprinted in 5 volumes, Dornach 1975.

Self-Education

13. Ralph Waldo Trine, *In Tune with the Infinite*, 1910.

14. See Rudolf Steiner's article on the Darwinist Bartholomäus Ritter von Carneri (1821–1909) in *Methodische Grundlagen der Anthroposophie, Gesammelte Aufsätze 1884–1901*, GA 30, pp. 452–61.

15. Schopenhauer, in Volume VII of his collected works, *Sämtliche Werke in XII Bänden*, with an introduction by Rudolf Steiner. 'Die beiden Grundprobleme der Ethik' in the chapter 'Metaphysische Grundlage', Stuttgart 1894.

16. Lessing, in *The Education of the Human Race* (1780) § 100.

For the Days of the Week

17. From *Seelenübungen I*, GA 267, pp. 68–73.

Sources

The following volumes are cited in this book. Where relevant, published editions of equivalent English translations are indicated. The works of Rudolf Steiner are listed with the volume numbers of the complete works in German, the *Gesamtausgabe* (GA), as published by Rudolf Steiner Verlag, Dornach, Switzerland.

RSP = Rudolf Steiner Press, UK
SB = SteinerBooks, USA

9   *Theosophy* (RSP/SB)

10 *Knowledge of the Higher Worlds/How to Know Higher Worlds* (RSP/SB)

34 *Lucifer-Gnosis; Grundlegende Aufsätze zur Anthroposophie und Berichte aus den Zeitschriften 'Luzifer' und 'Lucifer–Gnosis' 1903–1908*

61 *Menschengeschichte im Lichte der Geistesforschung*

107 *Disease, Karma and Healing* (RSP)

130 *Esoteric Christianity* (RSP)

134 *The World of the Senses and the World of the Spirit* (RSP)

143 *Erfahrungen des Übersinnlichen. Die drei Wege der Seele zu Christus*

177 *The Fall of the Spirits of Darkness* (RSP)

267 *Soul Exercises 1904–1924* (SB)

295 *Discussions with Teachers* (SB)

301 *The Renewal of Education* (SB)

310 *Human Values in Education* (SB)

All English-language titles are available via Rudolf Steiner Press, UK (www.rudolfsteinerpress.com) or SteinerBooks, USA (www.steinerbooks.org)